THE ROCKY MOUNTAIN REGION

The Rocky Mountains, commonly known as the Rockies, are a major mountain range in western North America. The Rockies stretch more than 3,000 miles (800 km) from northern British Columbia in western Canada to New Mexico in the southwestern United States. There are 10 distinct forests in the Rockies ranging from the dry southwestern forests of pinyon and ponderosa pines, oaks and junipers to the wetter northern forests dominated by Douglas-firs, hemlocks, white and lodgepole pines, aspens and firs. Each forest harbors its own distinctive array of edible plants.

There are a few simple rules one should follow when harvesting edible plants:

1. Ensure you are able to positively identify edible species. The rule of thumb is, "When in doubt, leave it out." To keep it simple, learn to identify 10 species that you know are common in the areas that you visit and that do not have poisonous mimics.
2. Be aware of the seasons during which different parts of the plants may be harvested.
3. Only collect plants that appear healthy.
4. Avoid areas that have been heavily sprayed with herbicides and polluted areas near roadways or factories.
5. Ensure it is legal to gather plants in the area.

Writer and bushcraft/survival specialist Jason Schwartz is the founder of Rocky Mountain Bushcraft, a blog that features articles, news stories, outdoor tips and product reviews written from a bushcraft and wilderness survival perspective. Schwartz is a former Red Cross certified Wilderness & Remote First Aid Instructor, and has taught bushcraft and wilderness survival techniques to a number of outdoor groups and organizations. He has also interned with the US Forest Service as a forestry technician and studied outdoor recreation, wilderness survival, forestry and wildland firefighting at Colorado Mountain College in Leadville, Colorado. In addition, Jason has written for magazines such as The New Pioneer and Backpacker, including writing the "Tinder Finder" portion of Backpacker's "Complete Guide to Fire," which won the 2015 National Magazine Award (NMA) in the Leisure Interests category. For more information, visit his blog at www.rockymountainbushcraft.co

Measurements depicted denote the height of plants unless otherwise indicated. Illustrations are not to scale.

N.B. – Many edible and medicinal wild plants have poisonous mimics. Never eat a wild plant or fruit unless you are absolutely sure it is safe to do so. The publisher makes no representation or warranties with respect to the accuracy, completeness, correctness or usefulness of this information and specifically disclaims any implied warranties of fitness for a particular purpose. The advice, strategies and/or techniques contained herein may not be suitable for all individuals. The publisher shall not be responsible for any physical harm (up to and including death), loss of profit or other commercial damage. The publisher assumes no liability brought or instituted by individuals or organizations arising out of or relating in any way to the application and/or use of the information, advice and strategies contained herein.

Waterford Press publishes reference guides to nature observation, outdoor recreation and survival skills. Product information is featured on the website:

www.waterfordpress.com

Text & illustrations © 2016, 2023 Waterford Press Inc. All rights reserved. Photos © Shutterstock. To order or for information on custom published products please call 800-434-2555 or email orderdesk@waterfordpress.com. For permissions or to share comments email editor@waterfordpress.com. 2309201

978-1-58355-976-5

$7.95 U.S.
$9.95 CAN

ISBN

50795

9 781583 559765

UPC

8 84682 00750 8

10 9 8 7 6 5 4 3 2 1   Made in the USA

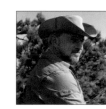

EDIBLE SURVIVAL PLANTS OF THE ROCKY MOUNTAINS

A Folding Pocket Guide to Familiar Species

SURVIVAL BASICS

Knowing which plant sources will satisfy your nutritional needs can help you in a survival situation. All food contains 4 basic components: protein, fat, carbohydrates and water.

Protein – Plant proteins are generally incomplete, meaning you need to combine more than one to get a whole protein. In a survival situation, you are unlikely to get much protein from plants, except from nuts and grains when you can find them.

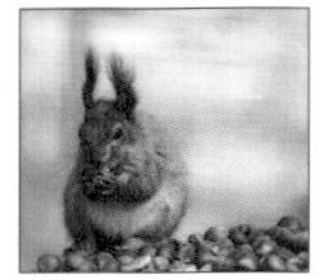

Fat – Nuts and seeds offer the greatest amount of fat, which aids digestion of protein and provides energy.

Carbohydrates – Two main types of carbs are sugar and starch. Plant sources for carbs include fruits, berries, stocks/stems/roots (including some barks), nuts and seeds.

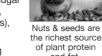

Nuts & seeds are the richest source of plant protein and fat.

Water – Essential to all body functions, including digestion. Water is contained in plant foods in varying quantities. When drinking water is not easily obtained, consider the caloric cost of digestion before consuming foods with low nutritional value (mushrooms) or high-calorie foods that have little water content and take longer to digest (nuts, seeds).

SAFETY FIRST

The most important consideration when finding wild plant food is to avoid poisoning from toxic plants. Some, like poison ivy, virgin's bowers and cow-parsnip, are **toxic when handled**, and can cause skin rashes and blistering. Other plants are **poisonous when eaten**.

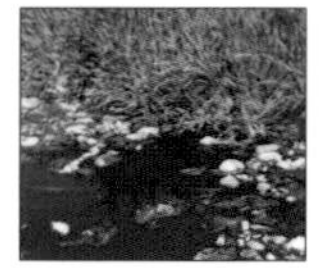

- Never collect plants growing in water that is contaminated or might contain parasites (like giardia).
- Some plants can develop fungal toxins – don't eat any fruit that shows signs of mildew or fungus.
- Signs of potentially poisonous plants include:

  - Milky sap
  - Bitter or soapy taste
  - Spines, thorns or fine hairs
  - Parsley or carrot-like foliage
  - Almond-scented

  - Leaves grow in threes
  - Grains with pink to blackish spurs
  - Seeds/beans inside pods

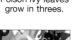

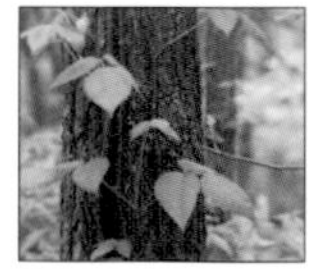

Never collect plants from contaminated water.

- The seeds of some plants, like chokecherry, contain cyanide and can kill you. Consider these general rules to determine if a berry is poisonous:

  - White, green and yellow berries are rarely edible.
  - 90% of blue, black and purple berries are edible.

  - 99% of druplet fruits (raspberries, blackberries, etc.) are edible.
  - Half of red berries are edible.

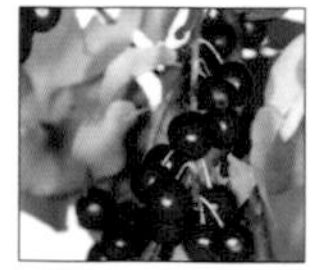

Poison ivy leaves grow in threes.

- Test all plant parts for edibility before you consume them. Some have both edible and inedible parts. Do not assume that a part that is edible when cooked is also edible when raw.
- Not all individuals react the same way to wild plants. Each person should test the plant part they are going to consume to ensure edibility and no reaction.
- Avoid wild mushrooms or any other fungi; it is difficult to distinguish between edible and toxic varieties and they have little nutritional value.

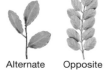

Chokecherry seeds contain cyanide.

HARVESTING TIPS

Fruits & Berries – A quick way to harvest fruit is to place a plastic sheet under a shrub or tree and shake it. Only ripe fruits will fall onto the sheet.

Leaves – Young leaves and shoots are generally tender and tastier. Older leaves are often tough and bitter.

Nuts & Seeds – To separate shells from nuts and seeds, chop up and immerse in water; the shells will float and the seeds will sink.

Removing Bitter Taste – Boil in several changes of water. To leach bitterness out, place leaves or fruits in a canvas bag and submerge in a clean stream or river for 1-3 days.

Drying – The key to drying plants is to do so slowly in a dry area, away from direct heat and sunlight. Hang plants upside down or place on raised screen and turn over occasionally. Slice or crush tubers and nut meats to speed up drying process.

TYPES OF EDIBLE WILD PLANTS

Stems & Leaves

   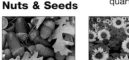

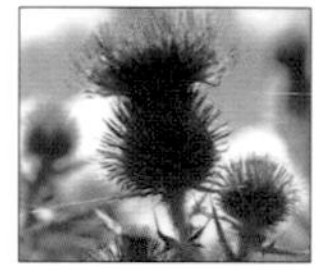

Shoots	Leaves	Pith	Cambium
Includes cattail, wild asparagus, and thistle.	Includes dandelion, dock, amaranth, plantain, onion, chicory, sorrel and lamb's quarter.	Growth inside plant stem is edible in cattails, thistle and burdock.	Inner layer between the bark and the wood is edible in many conifers, birch, poplar, aspen.

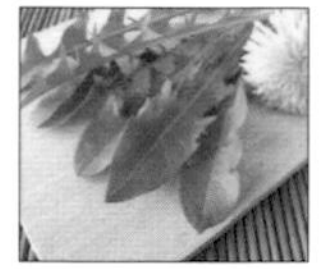

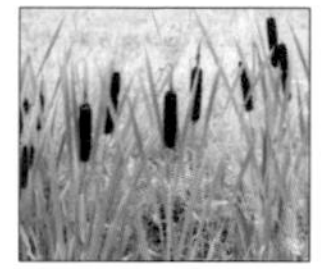

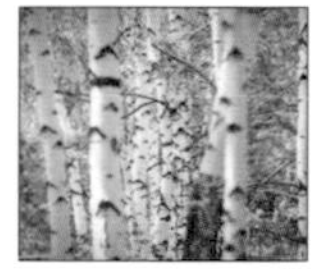

Nuts & Seeds

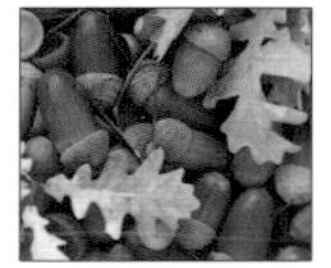

Acorns	Wild Sunflower	Hazelnuts	Pine Nuts
			Small seed kernels are located under cone scales.

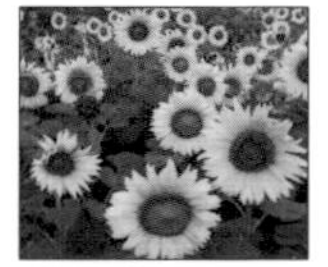

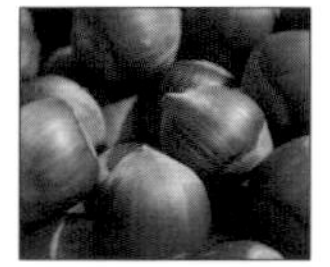

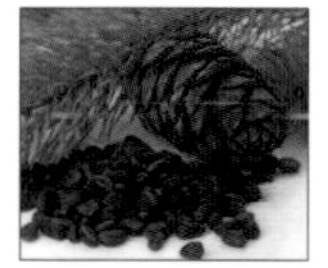

Fruits & Berries

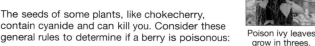 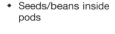

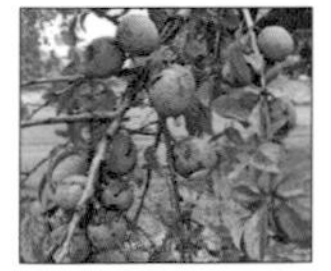

Wild Plum	Wild Red Raspberry	Rose Hips	Elderberry

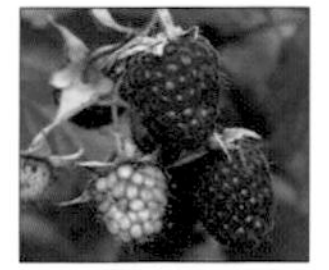

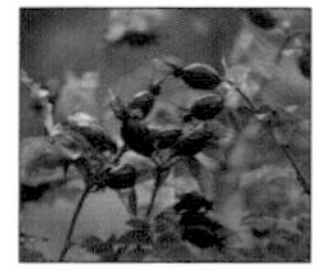

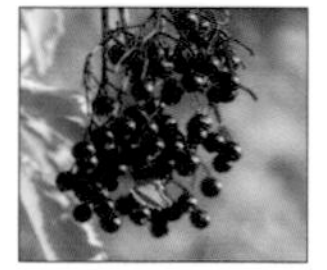

Roots & Tubers

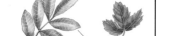 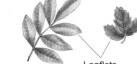 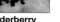

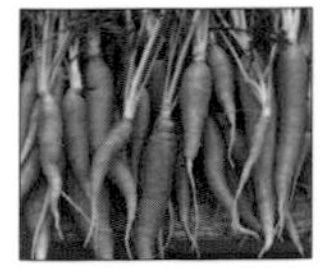

Taproot	Tuber	Bulb	Rhizome
Straight tapering root that grows downward.	An enlarged plant root.	An enlarged fleshy root of modified leaves.	A plant stem that sends out roots from its nodes.

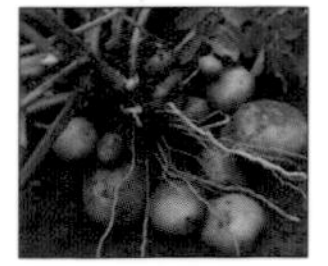

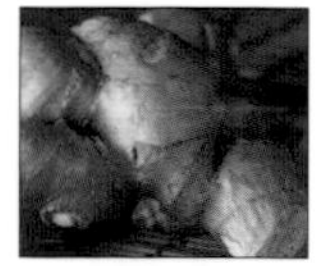

UNIVERSAL EDIBILITY TEST

This edibility test is best done while learning about the plant species, rather than in a survival situation. Practice with known edible plants that you can obtain (don't use plants treated with fertilizers or from roadsides or other polluted areas).

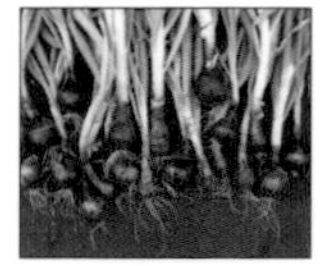

1. **Separate the plant into its components:** leaves, stems, roots, buds/seeds/nuts/fruits/flowers. Test one plant part at a time.
2. **Smell the plant for strong or repellent odors.** Remember that the smell of almonds indicates the likelihood of a cyanide compound and should be avoided.
3. **Test for contact poisoning** by placing the plant piece that you are testing on the inside of your elbow or wrist. Usually you will see a reaction within 15 minutes.
4. **Select a small portion of the plant and prepare it the way you intend to eat it.** Before placing it in your mouth, do another safety check and touch a small portion to the outside of your lip to see if you react with burning or itching.
5. **If no reaction on the lip after 3 minutes,** hold a small amount in your mouth for 15 minutes (do not swallow it).
6. **If no itching, burning, swelling, numbing** or other irritation after 15 minutes, you can assume you have no reaction.
7. **If any reaction occurs,** induce vomiting immediately.
8. **If no ill effects after 8 hours, eat a small amount.** Wait another 8 hours and if no reaction, consider the food palatable to you.

Edible Plant Myths

- "If animals can eat it, so can I." — Not true.
- "Boiling a plant in water will remove toxins." — Not always so. If you have to eat it, follow the universal edibility test rules.
- "Plants with red parts are poisonous." — Not always true, learn to identify plants.

PLANT IDENTIFICATION

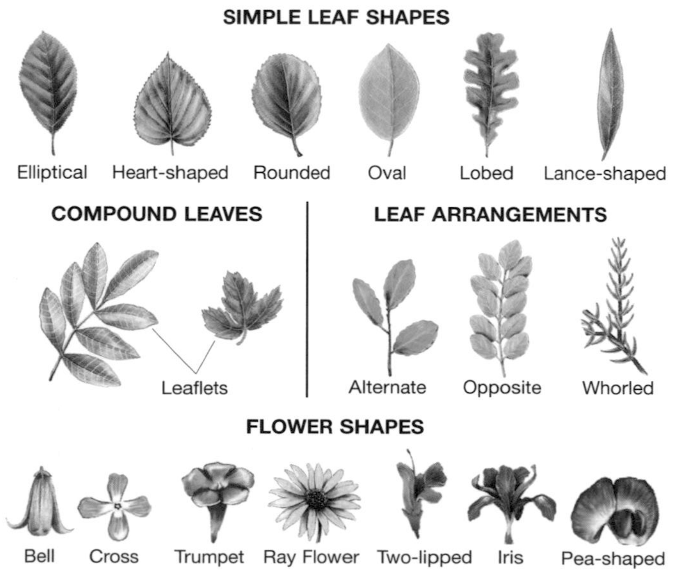

SIMPLE LEAF SHAPES

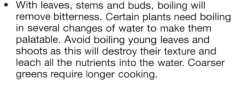

Elliptical   Heart-shaped   Rounded   Oval   Lobed   Lance-shaped

COMPOUND LEAVES

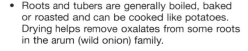

Leaflets

LEAF ARRANGEMENTS

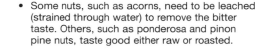

Alternate   Opposite   Whorled

FLOWER SHAPES

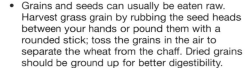
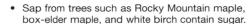

Bell   Cross   Trumpet   Ray Flower   Two-lipped   Iris   Pea-shaped

---

PREPARING WILD EDIBLES

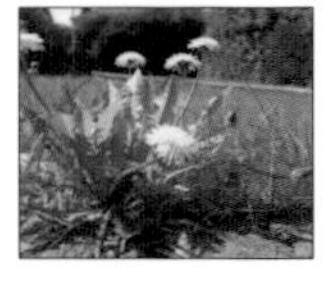

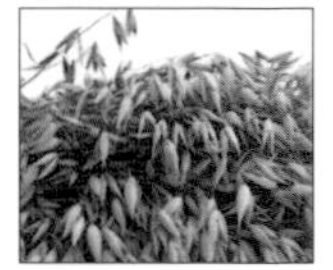

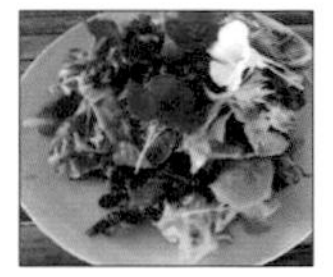

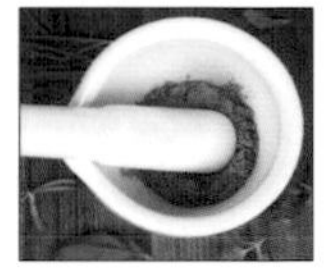

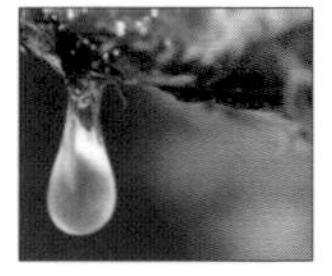

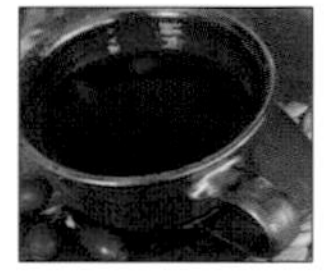

As you learn to identify the plant species, also learn how to prepare them for maximum nutritional benefit. Generally, plant food is prepared in one of the following ways: soaking, boiling, cooking, drying, or leaching. While some plants can be eaten raw, others must be cooked to make them edible or to remove an unappealing or bitter taste.

- With leaves, stems and buds, boiling will remove bitterness. Certain plants need boiling in several changes of water to make them palatable. Avoid boiling young leaves and shoots as this will destroy their texture and leach all the nutrients into the water. Coarser greens require longer cooking.

- Roots and tubers are generally boiled, baked or roasted and can be cooked like potatoes. Drying helps remove oxalates from some roots in the arum (wild onion) family.

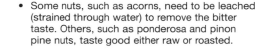

- Some nuts, such as acorns, need to be leached (strained through water) to remove the bitter taste. Others, such as ponderosa and pinon pine nuts, taste good either raw or roasted.

- Grains and seeds can usually be eaten raw. Harvest grass grain by rubbing the seed heads between your hands or pound them with a rounded stick; toss the grains in the air to separate the wheat from the chaff. Dried grains should be ground up for better digestibility.

To extract maximum nutrients from plants, grind them into a pulp.

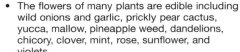

- Sap from trees such as Rocky Mountain maple, box-elder maple, and white birch contain sugar.

- The flowers of many plants are edible including wild onions and garlic, prickly pear cactus, yucca, mallow, pineapple weed, dandelions, chicory, clover, mint, rose, sunflower, and violets.

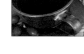

- Teas are made by steeping one handful of leaves (or needles), stems or fruits in 2 cups of hot water (preferably covered) for 10 minutes. Do not boil. Steeping the tea longer will enhance the strength of the tea. When certain roots and bark are used in tea, they should be shredded or crushed thoroughly before steeping. Two very nutritious teas high in vitamin C can be made from pine needles and rose hips (the rounded fruits of rose bushes).

The Importance of Charcoal

Charcoal is a valuable resource in the case of accidental poisoning. Ground-up charcoal in water will induce vomiting when swallowed. The residual charcoal left in the stomach will absorb the remaining toxins in the stomach. If you suspect poisoning seek medical attention as soon as possible.

Ponderosa Pine
Pinus ponderosa
To 268 ft. (82 m)

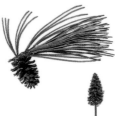

Description: Large coniferous tree with evergreen needles 4-10 in. (10-25 cm) long, usually in bundles of three. Bark orange-brown to cinnamon on mature trees with jigsaw-like plates outlined by deep, black fissures. Immature trees have light gray to brown bark. Cones are oval, 3-5 in. (8-14 cm) long, thick, with spine-tipped scales.
Habitat: Plains to Montane Zone. Southern British Columbia to New Mexico.
Harvest: Nuts, inner bark (cambium) and needles.
Preparation: Inner bark can be eaten raw year round and tastes similar to sheep's fat. To harvest, use a knife with a baton (an arm's length branch used as a mallet to pound the back of the knife) to remove bark from tree. Scrape the thin white layer from inner bark. This can be eaten raw, roasted, boiled, or fried.
Nuts: Ponderosa pines produce large edible nuts inside their green cones during late summer and autumn. To access the nuts, split the green cone 4 ways using a knife and baton or axe/hatchet or smash green cones with a rock until they are soft enough to pull apart, allowing you to access the nuts. You can also roast the cones over a fire until they open and release the nuts.
Comments: The ponderosa pine holds the distinction of being the world's tallest pine tree, with the tallest recorded example coming in at 268.5 ft. (81.8 m) tall.

Pinon Pine
Pinus edulis
To 45 ft. (13.7 m)

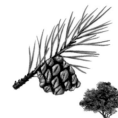

Description: Coniferous, bushy evergreen tree with long 1-2 in. (3-5 cm) needles that usually come in bundles of two. Typically reaches only 20-30 ft. high at maturity. Trunk is often crooked. Bark is reddish to yellow-brown, irregularly furrowed and scaly. Cones are globular/spherical, 1.2 to 2 in. (3-5 cm) long and somewhat similar in appearance to ponderosa pine cones. Often found growing alongside junipers.
Identification Tip: There are several ways to distinguish a pinon pine from a ponderosa pine. First, pinon is shorter and "bushier." Second, its needles are bundled in twos. Third, dried pinon resin has a unique scent like incense.
Habitat: Foothills to Montane zones, often mixed with junipers. Southwestern Wyoming, Utah, Southern Colorado and New Mexico.
Harvest: Nuts, needles, inner bark.
Preparation: Nuts: Pinon pines produce large, edible nuts in their cones in autumn. To access the nuts, pull them directly from the cones or roast over a fire until they open, releasing the nuts. Inner bark (cambium) can be eaten in an emergency if fried, roasted or boiled.
Comments: Pinon pine nuts were once a vital food source to Native Americans.

Gambel Oak (Scrub Oak)
Quercus gambelii
To 30 ft. (9 m)

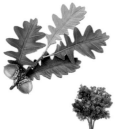

Description: Short, scraggly, scrubby deciduous oak tree with classic oak leaf shape. Bears large acorns. Leaves are generally 3-5 in. (7-12 cm) long and 2-4 in. (4-6 cm) wide, deeply lobed on each side of the central vein; the upper surface is glossy and dark green, the undersurface is paler and velvety. Acorns mature in September, turning from green to golden brown.
Habitat: Foothills to Montane Zone. From Southern Wyoming to Utah, Colorado and New Mexico.
Harvest: Nut meats from acorns.
Preparation: Remove nut meat and soak for multiple hours in several changes of water until bitter taste is removed. Put nut meat in a cloth bag and soak in a stream, lake or river. Nut meat can be eaten raw after soaking *only* if potable water was used. Otherwise, boil it first to remove any pathogens.
Comments: Acorns from gambel oak trees were a vital food source for Native American tribes. The wood of gambel oak is hard and strong like eastern oak trees, making it excellent for cooking, smoking, or constructing primitive tools.

Rocky Mountain Douglas-Fir
Pseudotsuga menziesii var. glauca
To 476 ft. (145 m)

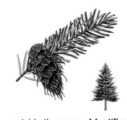

Description: Coniferous evergreen with spreading branches. Adult trees have open crowns. Bark on young trees: thin and smooth with resin blisters. Bark on mature trees: ridged and fissured. Needles are flat and blunt, .75-1.25 in. (2-3 cm) long, spirally arranged, often twisted into 2 rows. Female seed cones are 2-4 in. (5-10 cm) long with distinctive 3-toothed bracts that project from the cone. These bracts look like streamers that hang slightly outside the cones. **Identification Tip:** Douglas-fir is often mistaken for spruce. The easiest way to identify it is by its highly distinctive cones. Another method is to grab the needles. If the needles feel hard, sharp and poke your skin, it is a spruce. Douglas-fir needles are much softer and will usually cause little to no discomfort when grabbed.
Habitat: Foothills to Subalpine Zones. British Columbia and Alberta to New Mexico.
Harvest: Inner bark, needles.
Uses: Inner bark (cambium) can be eaten raw year round. *Fir needle tea:* Steep needles in boiling water for a vitamin C rich tea. **WARNING:** Due to the resin content, large amounts of fir tea can be toxic. Pregnant women should never consume fir tea.
Comments: Beautiful, majestic and long-lived, Douglas-firs have been known to survive up to (1,300 years.

Skunkbush/Squawbush/Three-Leaved Sumac
Rhus trilobata
To 6 ft. (1.8 m)

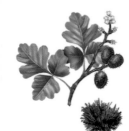

Description: Tall, woody, perennial shrub. Leaves are lobed and grow in 3s. Leaves look similar to small oak leaves and are sometimes mistaken for poison oak. Leaves have a strong, skunk-like odor, especially when crushed. You will know a skunkbush by the distinctive odor when you walk close to one. Berries are bunched in dense clusters and are red, sticky, fuzzy and hard to the touch. They have a strong lemony flavor that is mildly tart/sweet.
Identification Tip: Skunkbush is easily distinguished from poison oak by its red berries; poison oak berries are greenish/white.
Habitat: Common throughout many areas of the Rockies. Plains to Montane Zones. Alberta to New Mexico.
Harvest: Berries.
Preparation: Berries can be eaten raw, dried, or cooked and are high in vitamin C. Berries can also be made into a lemonade-like drink by straining warm water through the berries into a container. Do not use hot water, as it will make the juice too sour/bitter. Berries can be dried and saved for later use.
Comments: Like wild rose hips, skunkbush berries are one of the few berries that can still be found during winter. Popping a few of them into your canteen is also a great way to add a pleasant taste to drinking water.

Chokecherry
Prunus virginiana var. melanocarpa
To 25 ft. (7.6 m)

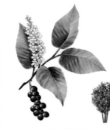

Description: Small deciduous tree or shrub. Bark is dark gray and smooth textured. Leaves are up to 4 in. (10.1 cm) long, ovate shaped and pointed, with tiny teeth that run along the entirety of the outside edge. Cylindrical clusters of spring flowers are succeeded by dark, red-purple berries.
Habitat: Plains to Montane zones. Alaska to New Mexico.
Harvest: Fruit.
Preparation: Edible, pea-sized fruits range from tart to sweet. **NOTE: ONLY black cherries are edible.** Fruit pits and leaves contain a weak cyanide that is destroyed by cooking or drying. Fruit is edible raw, but make sure to spit out the seeds. **CAUTION: Do not eat any other part of the plant, including light colored/green cherries, as they are poisonous.**
Comments: Despite their uninviting name and occasional mouth-puckering quality, most chokecherries are quite tasty, ranging from a mild bittersweet flavor to as sweet as a domestic black cherry. Chokecherries were used by Native Americans to make pemmican. Chokecherry wood is a hardwood similar to the wood of the eastern black cherry, making it good for smoking meat or for making primitive bows, arrows or tools.

Wild Wax Currant
Ribes spp./R. cereum
To 6 ft. (1.8 m)

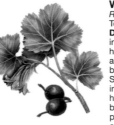

Description: Leaves are small, ranging from .5-1.63 in. (1-4 cm), and are kidney or fan-shaped. Leaves have a distinct pleasant smell as if walking through a fruit farm. White to pink flowers are succeeded by red currants. Berries ripen between July and September depending on the altitude. Berries range in color from bright orange-red to crimson red and are covered with barbed spines. Berries ripen in late summer and autumn. They are typically pink or red when ripe but can also be yellow or purple.
Habitat: Dry slopes, Plains to Subalpine Zones. British Columbia to New Mexico.
Harvest: Fruit, flowers.
Preparation: Berries are edible raw or cooked. Due to their high pectin content, they are great for making pies or jellies. Flowers can be eaten raw. Large quantities of raw wax currants can cause stomach aches in people with sensitive stomachs. Boil them before eating large quantities to avoid discomfort. The boiling water also brings out the pectin and makes the berries taste sweeter.
Comments: One of the most abundant and widespread berries in the Rockies during late summer. Wax currants were used by Native Americans to make pemmican.

Common Bearberry (Kinnikinnick)
Arctostaphylos uva-ursi
To 12 in. (30 cm)

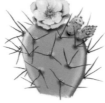

Description: Small evergreen groundcover shrub. In many areas of the Rockies it literally carpets the forest floor. Leaves are dark green in color. Leaves are small, shiny, stiff and spoon-shaped. Small .13-.25 in. white or pinkish flowers appear in May to June and produce mealy, .25-.38 in. (6-10 mm) bright red berries by late summer.
Habitat: Foothills to Alpine Zones. Alaska to New Mexico.
Harvest: Fruit.
Preparation: Berries are edible raw or cooked. Raw bearberries are mealy and range from tasteless to mildly sweet. Bearberries can often be found during winter, even underneath several feet of snow. **WARNING:** Bearberries can cause liver damage from extended use (more than three days) due to their high tannin and arbutin content. To avoid this issue, boil them, which also makes the berries sweeter.
Comments: Native tribes of the west smoked dried bearberry leaves when tobacco was unavailable. Bearberries were also used by Native Americans to make pemmican. The bearberry plant gets its name because bears are thought to be fond of eating its berries.

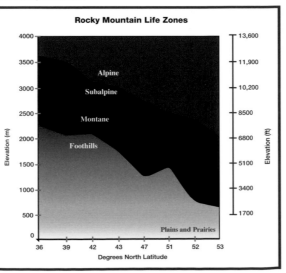

Rocky Mountain Life Zones

(chart: Elevation in meters and feet vs. Degrees North Latitude, showing zones: Alpine, Subalpine, Montane, Foothills, Plains and Prairies)

Prickly Pear Cactus
Opuntia spp.
Pads to 2-12 in. (5-30 cm)

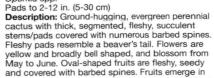 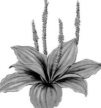

Description: Ground-hugging, evergreen perennial cactus with thick, segmented, fleshy, succulent pads covered with numerous barbed spines. Fleshy pads resemble a beaver's tail. Flowers are yellow and broadly bell shaped, and blossom from May to June. Oval-shaped fruits are fleshy, seedy and covered with barbed spines. Fruits emerge in late summer and autumn. They are typically pink or red when ripe but can also be yellow or purple.
Habitat: High Mountain Deserts and Prairies up to Montane Zones. Lower British Columbia and Alberta to New Mexico.
Harvest: Fleshy pads, fruits and flowers.
Preparation: To prepare the fleshy pads, burn off large spines. Small spines will remain; take a knife and carefully cut off outer skin to remove remaining spines. Flesh can be eaten raw, roasted, or boiled and has a taste similar to cucumber. To eat the fruits, prepare in the same manner. Fruits are delicious and can be eaten raw as well. Flowers are delicious and can be eaten raw as well.
CAUTION: The smallest spines are hard to see. Despite their small size, they can cause aggravating skin wounds for days. While removing spines, use a sharpened branch, heavy gloves, heavy cloth or animal skin to hold cactus pads. If you do get barbed, lightly scrape skin with a knife to remove as many barbs as possible. **NEVER** attempt to remove spines with your mouth. They could work their way into your tongue or windpipe, causing extreme discomfort or even serious injury or death.
Comments: Despite the risk of the prickly pear's spines, if reasonable caution is used, they are an excellent survival food that is widely available in many areas.

Cattail
Typha latifolia
To 7 ft. (2.1 m)

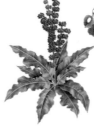

Description: Large upright herb has long, swordlike leaves sheathing the base of the stem. Tiny flowers bloom in a long terminal cluster and are succeeded by downy brownish seeds.
Habitat: Plains to Montane Zones from Southern Yukon to New Mexico.
Harvest: Shoots, roots, stalks, spikes.
Preparation: Young shoots can be eaten raw. Stalks can be peeled and boiled until tender. Green seed heads can be boiled and eaten like corn on the cob.
CAUTION: Cattail down is an excellent insulation material that can be stuffed into shoes, jacket, gloves, or sleeping bag to provide warmth in a survival situation.

Stinging Nettle
Urtica gracilis
To 6 ft. (1.8 m)

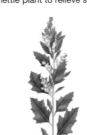

Description: Erect, leafy plant is covered with stinging hairs that cause a burning sensation. Leaves are long, thin and deeply serrated. Stem is somewhat square. Flowers are greenish and hang in clusters along the upper stem. **Identification Tip:** Often mistaken for wild mint due to its appearance. The easiest way to identify nettle is the lack of a mint smell as well as the stinging hairs that cover the stems and leaves, which mint does not have.
Habitat: Plains, Foothills and Montane Zones.
Harvest: Leaves, young shoots.
Preparation: WARNING: Stings can cause rash, hives or allergic reactions. They can also cause uterine contractions. Pregnant women should avoid this plant. To make the plant safe to eat, boil, steam or dry nettle leaves or shoots before eating them to neutralize the stinging acid. Young leaves are best, but mature leaves may be eaten as well. **TIP:** To prevent stings while harvesting, use mullein leaves, a heavy piece of cloth/bandana or coat your hands with mud. If stung, rub the crushed leaves of curly dock, plantain or yarrow on the affected area to relieve symptoms. Despite the difficulties in dealing with their stinging hairs, nettle is a delicious and highly nutritious food source with a taste like spinach.
Comments: Dried nettle leaves contain up to 40% protein, one of the highest in the plant kingdom.

Plantain
Plantago major
To 12 in. (30 cm)

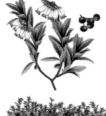

Description: Common weed. Basal leaves have wavy edges and parallel veins. Greenish flowers have purplish anthers and bloom in long spikes.
Habitat: Plains to Montane Zones. Alaska to New Mexico.
Harvest: Leaves, seeds.
Preparation: Eat leaves raw or boiled or steep to make tea. Strip seeds from flower stalks and boil them or dry them and grind into flour. Young flower stalks can be boiled and eaten.
Comments: Rich in vitamins A, C and minerals. The crushed leaves of plantain can be applied to the sting from a nettle plant to relieve symptoms.

Curly Dock
Rumex crispus
To 4 ft. (1.2 m)

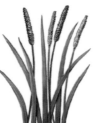

Description: Common perennial weed with jointed stems. Large leaves have curled or wavy edges that can be up to 12 in. long (30.4 cm). Smaller leaves alternate along stem. Flowers have no petals and are succeeded by small, heart-shaped winged seeds that turn a deep, rusty red color later in the season.
Habitat: Plains to Montane Zones on disturbed ground. Alaska to New Mexico.
Harvest: Young leaves, seeds.
Preparation: Young leaves are best. Boil in two changes of water to remove excess oxalic acid before eating. As long as the leaves are leached and cooked, they make a tasty cooked vegetable, comparable to kale. Seeds are bitter but edible. Boil them in several changes of water before eating.
Comments: The crushed leaves of curly dock can be applied to the sting from a nettle plant to relieve symptoms.

Lamb's Quarters/Wild Spinach
Chenopodium album
To 8 ft. (2.4 m)

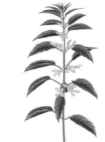

Description: Erect grayish-green colored annual herb. Leaves are toothed and triangular in appearance and are compared to a goose's foot or spearhead. Leaves alternate along stem and are whitish cast to the touch. Both leaves and stems have a whitish cast. Flowers form green clumps at the junctions of leaves and stems which produce many seeds. **CAUTION:** Do not eat plants in this family if they have a rank smell or bad taste.
Habitat: Disturbed ground. Plains to Subalpine Zones. Alaska to New Mexico.
Harvest: All parts of the plant are edible.
Preparation: Leaves, stalks and seeds are edible raw or cooked. If eaten raw, young leaves taste best. High in vitamins A and C, seeds can be ground into flour or used whole in soups and stews. **CAUTION:** Eating large amounts of raw lamb's quarters can cause mild oxilate/nitrate poisoning. It is ok to eat in smaller quantities, but best to boil first if you plan to eat larger quantities (strain out water before eating which contains the excess oxalates).
Comments: Young, raw lamb's quarters leaves are mild and delicious and are considered by many to be superior in flavor to domestic spinach.

Burdock
Arctium spp.
To 6 ft. (1.8 m)

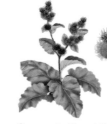

Description: Large herb has a basal rosette of 2-5 very large leaves up to 28 in. (70 cm) long. Alternate leaves are green above and woolly below. Large lower leaves are heart-shaped. Pink to purple flowers bloom in clusters at the base of the leaves.
Identification Tip: A square stem and strong minty smell are the easiest way to identify this plant. If it smells like mint, it is mint.
Habitat: Disturbed areas, fields, vacant lots.
Harvest: Roots, leafstalks, young leaves.
Preparation: Peel roots and boil in 2 changes of water. Peel young stalks and eat like celery. Eat young leaves raw or boiled.
Comments: The prickly heads (burrs) of this plant attach readily to fur, feathers and clothing and aid in seed dispersal. The burrs were the inspiration for Velcro.

Thistle
Cirsium spp.
To 6 ft. (1.8 m)

Description: Erect, tall weed with stems, leaves and branches covered with sharp spines. Leaves are grayish-green in color and deeply lobed. Spear-shaped, toothy leaves are up to 5-10 in. long (15-25 cm). First-year plants form rosettes. Second-year plants grow a flowering stalk with alternate leaves. Pink-purple flowers appear between June and August depending on elevation.
Habitat: Plains to Subalpine Zones. Alaska to New Mexico.
Harvest: Roots, leaves, young stalks, seeds.
Preparation: Leaves can be rendered palatable by carefully stripping off the spines. Eat raw or cook as a vegetable. Peel young stalks and eat raw like celery or cook like asparagus. Thistle seeds can be ground into flour. Immature flower heads can be eaten raw, steamed or fried. Roots can be eaten roasted or boiled. Seeds can be eaten roasted.
Comments: The down from thistle flowers makes an excellent flash tinder. Thistle down burns quickly; be sure to have a tinder bundle of dry grasses, dead pine needles, inner bark, etc., ready to catch the flame.

Wild Rose
Rosa spp.
To 8 ft. (2.4 m)

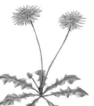

Description: Perennial shrub with reddish colored stems and branches covered with thorns. The leaves are ovate shaped, toothed, and 1-1.5 in. (2.5-3.8 cm) long. Flowers are succeeded by fruits called hips that are rich in vitamin C.
Habitat: Plains to Subalpine zones. From Alaska to New Mexico.
Harvest: Fruit, flower petals.
Preparation: Eat petals and hips raw or brewed in tea. The flavor of hips ranges from bland to mildly sweet. Boiling makes them sweeter and more palatable. Seeds are considered mildly poisonous; it's best to spit them out when eating raw hips to destroy the poisonous compounds.
Comments: Just one rose hip contains roughly 500 mg of vitamin C. Rose hips are one of the few fruits still available during the winter months, making them a good survival food when other food sources might be scarce.

Dandelion
Taraxacum officinale
To 16 in. (40.6 cm)

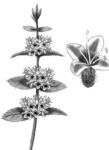

Description: Long leaves are all basal and irregularly toothed. Puffy yellow flowerheads are succeeded by plume-tailed seeds that are spread by the wind.
Habitat: Plains to Montane Zones. Alaska to New Mexico.
Harvest: All parts of the plant are edible.
Preparation: Leaves can be used in salads or as a potherb. Dried flowers can be steeped to make tea. The root can be prepared like carrots or dried and crushed to make a coffee substitute.
Comments: A rich source of vitamin A. The plant's coarsely toothed leaves give the plant its name, which means lion's tooth.

Wild Mint
Mentha spp.
To 32 in. (80 cm)

Description: Opposite leaves grow along square stems. Small, bell-shaped, pink, lilac or white flowers bloom in clusters at the base of the leaves.
Identification Tip: A square stem and strong minty smell are the easiest way to identify this plant. If it smells like mint, it is mint.
Habitat: Plains to Montane Zones. Alaska to New Mexico.
Harvest: Leaves and flower buds.
Preparation: Eat raw or boiled or use to make wild mint tea.
Comments: Leaves have strong minty, bitter flavor and are a seasoning for meat.